A Love's Labor:

The Dementia Caregiver's Guide

Introduction

A Love's Labor: The Dementia Caregiver's Guide is an invaluable resource for those caring for loved ones with dementia. This comprehensive guide offers practical strategies, emotional support, and expert insights to navigate the challenges of this journey. Discover essential information about dementia, learn effective caregiving techniques, and find the strength and resilience to provide exceptional care while preserving your own well-being.

This book is your trusted companion, offering hope, support, and practical guidance every step of the way.

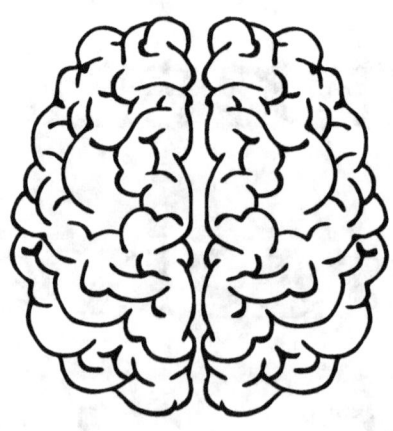

Contents

Part I: Understanding Dementia

Chapter 1: What is Dementia?

Chapter 2: The Psychology of Dementia

Chapter 3: Diagnosing Dementia

Part II: Navigating the Dementia Journey

Chapter 4: Managing the Early Stages

Chapter 5: Understanding Brain Disorders

1. Alcohol and Dementia
2. Alzheimer's Disease
3. Amnestic Mild Cognitive Impairment
4. Cerebral Amyloid Angiopathy
5. Neuroplasticity and Dementia
6. Neurotransmitters and Dementia
7. Electrical Signaling and Dementia

Chapter 6: Medical Care and Management

1. Evaluating the Person with Dementia
2. Medical Treatment and Management
3. Common Medical Challenges (pain, dehydration, pneumonia, constipation, vision problems, etc.)

Contents

Chapter 7: Prevention and Symptom Management

1. Preventing Dementia
2. Decreasing Dementia Symptoms
3. Managing Memory Problems

Part III: Caring for the Caregiver

Chapter 8: Prioritizing Self-Care

1. The Impact of Caregiving
2. Caregiver Burnout
3. Preparing for the Caregiving Journey
4. Maintaining Physical and Mental Health
5. Building Resilience
6. Managing Emotional Reactions

Chapter 9: Practical Caregiving Strategies

1. Building Strong Connections
2. Care Planning and Coordination
3. In-Home and Long-Term Care Options
4. Adapting to Daily Life Changes
5. Managing Mood Swings
6. Addressing Sleep Disturbances
7. Stress Management Techniques
8. Managing Behavioral Challenges

Contents

Part IV: Additional Considerations

Chapter 10: Legal and Financial Planning

Chapter 11: Effective Communication Strategies

Chapter 12: The Importance of Respite Care

Chapter 13: End-of-Life Care and Planning

Part I: Understanding Dementia
Chapter 1: What is Dementia?

Dementia is a general term for a decline in mental ability that interferes with daily life. It's not a specific disease but rather a group of symptoms caused by various brain disorders.

Key characteristics of dementia include:

- Memory loss: Difficulty remembering recent events, names, or appointments.

- Difficulty with thinking and problem-solving: Struggling with tasks that were once routine, like balancing a checkbook or following a recipe.

- Challenges with language: Trouble finding the right words, understanding what others are saying, or expressing thoughts clearly.

- Changes in mood and behavior: Experiencing mood swings, becoming easily agitated or withdrawn.

- Problems with spatial awareness: Difficulty judging distances, understanding spatial relationships, or getting lost in familiar places.

It's important to note that dementia is not a normal part of aging, and while it primarily affects older adults, it can occur in younger people.

Part I: Understanding Dementia
Chapter 1: What is Dementia?

Types of Dementia

While dementia is an umbrella term, several specific conditions can cause it. Here are some common types:

- **Alzheimer's disease:** The most common form, characterized by gradual memory loss and cognitive decline.

- **Vascular dementia:** Caused by damage to blood vessels in the brain, often linked to stroke or high blood pressure.

- **Lewy body dementia:** Involves abnormal protein deposits in the brain, leading to fluctuations in cognitive abilities, visual hallucinations, and movement difficulties.

- **Frontotemporal dementia:** Affects the frontal and temporal lobes of the brain, resulting in changes in personality, behavior, and language.

- **Mixed dementia:** A combination of different types of dementia, often Alzheimer's and vascular dementia.

Part I: Understanding Dementia
Chapter 1: What is Dementia?

The Progression of Dementia

Dementia is a progressive disease, meaning it worsens over time. The rate of progression varies widely between individuals. Generally, it's divided into stages:

- **Early-stage dementia:** Mild memory loss, difficulty with complex tasks, and changes in mood or behavior.

- **Middle-stage dementia:** Increasing memory loss, challenges with daily living activities, and more pronounced behavioral changes.

- **Late-stage dementia:** Severe memory loss, loss of ability to communicate, and dependence on others for basic care.

The Impact of Dementia

Dementia not only affects the individual but also has a profound impact on families and caregivers. It can lead to emotional stress, financial burdens, and challenges in maintaining relationships.

Part I: Understanding Dementia
Chapter 2: The Psychology of Dementia

Dementia is not just a physical decline; it profoundly impacts the mind and emotions of those affected. Understanding the psychological aspects of dementia is crucial for caregivers and loved ones to provide effective support.

Emotional Changes

One of the most noticeable impacts of dementia is on emotional regulation. Individuals with dementia may experience:

- Mood swings: Rapid shifts from happiness to sadness or anger.

- Anxiety and agitation: Feelings of unease, restlessness, or irritability.

- Depression: A persistent low mood, loss of interest in activities, and feelings of hopelessness.

- Apathy: A lack of motivation or interest in previously enjoyed activities.

Part I: Understanding Dementia
Chapter 2: The Psychology of Dementia

It's important to remember that these emotional changes are often a result of the brain's deterioration and not intentional behavior.

Cognitive Changes

Beyond memory loss, dementia affects other cognitive functions, leading to:

- Disorientation: Difficulty recognizing places, people, or time.

- Delusions and hallucinations: False beliefs or perceptions.

- Personality changes: Shifts in behavior, becoming more withdrawn, suspicious, or aggressive.

These changes can be challenging for both the person with dementia and their caregivers.

Impact on Self-Esteem and Identity

As dementia progresses, individuals may experience a decline in self-esteem and a loss of identity. They may feel frustrated, helpless, or ashamed due to their increasing dependence on others.

Part I: Understanding Dementia
Chapter 2: The Psychology of Dementia

The Caregiver's Perspective

Caregivers also face significant psychological challenges. They may experience:

- Stress and burnout: The demands of caregiving can be overwhelming.

- Guilt and frustration: Feelings of inadequacy or anger towards the person with dementia.

- Grief and loss: As the disease progresses, caregivers may experience a sense of loss as the person they knew changes.

Understanding the psychological aspects of dementia is essential for providing compassionate and effective care. It helps caregivers to respond with empathy and patience, creating a supportive environment for the person with dementia.

Part I: Understanding Dementia
Chapter 3: Diagnosing Dementia

Diagnosing dementia can be a complex process as there's no single definitive test. It often involves a combination of assessments and tests conducted by healthcare professionals.

The Diagnostic Process

1. **Medical History and Physical Exam:**
   - A comprehensive review of the patient's medical history, including symptoms, medications, and family history of dementia.
   - A physical examination to rule out other potential causes of cognitive decline, such as thyroid problems, vitamin deficiencies, or infections.
2. **Cognitive Assessment:**
   - A series of tests to evaluate memory, language, problem-solving, and other cognitive functions.
   - Common tests include the Mini-Mental State Examination (MMSE) and the Clock Drawing Test.
3. **Neurological Examination:**
   - Assessing motor skills, reflexes, coordination, and balance to identify any neurological issues.
4. **Laboratory Tests:**
   - Blood tests to rule out other medical conditions that might mimic dementia symptoms.
5. **Brain Imaging:**
   - Techniques like CT scans, MRI scans, or PET scans to visualize the brain structure and identify abnormalities.

Part I: Understanding Dementia
Chapter 3: Diagnosing Dementia

6. Cerebrospinal Fluid (CSF) Analysis:
- In some cases, a lumbar puncture may be performed to analyze the cerebrospinal fluid for biomarkers of certain types of dementia, such as Alzheimer's disease.

Challenges in Diagnosis

- Early-stage dementia: Symptoms may be subtle, making it difficult to distinguish from normal aging.
- Differential diagnosis: Other conditions like depression, anxiety, or sleep disorders can mimic dementia symptoms.
- Access to specialized care: Availability of neurologists and dementia specialists may vary.

Accurate and timely diagnosis is crucial for initiating appropriate treatment, providing support, and planning for the future.

Part II: Navigating the Dementia Journey
Chapter 4: Managing the Early Stages

The early stages of dementia can be a challenging time for both the person with dementia and their caregivers. However, with the right strategies, it's possible to maintain a good quality of life.

Key Strategies for Early-Stage Dementia

- Open Communication: Discuss the diagnosis openly with the person with dementia and their family. This helps to build trust and create a supportive environment.

- Safety Measures: Assess the home for potential hazards and make necessary adjustments. Install safety features like grab bars, non-slip mats, and adequate lighting.

- Memory Aids: Utilize tools like calendars, reminders, and note-taking to help with daily tasks and appointments.
- Maintain a Routine: Consistent daily routines can provide a sense of security and reduce confusion.

- Physical and Mental Stimulation: Encourage activities like puzzles, games, or hobbies to stimulate the mind. Regular exercise is also beneficial for both physical and mental health.

- Social Interaction: Maintaining social connections is essential for emotional well-being. Encourage participation in social activities and support groups.

Part II: Navigating the Dementia Journey
Chapter 4: Managing the Early Stages

- Caregiver Support: Seek support from family, friends, or support groups. It's crucial to take care of your own well-being as a caregiver.

Addressing Challenges

- Memory Loss: Use simple language and avoid overwhelming the person with too much information.

- Mood Changes: Create a calm and predictable environment. Be patient and understanding.

- Difficulty with Daily Tasks: Break down tasks into smaller steps and provide clear instructions. Offer assistance when needed without taking over.

Remember: Early intervention and support can significantly improve the quality of life for both the person with dementia and their caregivers. It's important to consult with healthcare professionals for personalized guidance.

Part II: Navigating the Dementia Journey
Chapter 4: Managing the Early Stages

The Importance of Maintaining Independence

One of the primary goals in the early stages of dementia is to help the individual maintain as much independence as possible. This can significantly improve their quality of life and sense of self-worth.

- Encouraging Self-Care: Assisting with personal hygiene tasks while promoting independence can be beneficial.

- Financial Management: Early planning and discussions about financial matters are crucial. Consider appointing a power of attorney or setting up a trust.

- Driving Safety: Assessing driving abilities and making necessary adjustments, such as limiting night driving or avoiding busy traffic, is essential.

Communication Strategies

Effective communication is vital in the early stages of dementia.

- Active Listening: Giving full attention to the person with dementia, maintaining eye contact, and using open-ended questions can facilitate understanding.

- Simplifying Language: Avoiding complex sentences and using clear, concise language can improve comprehension.

Part II: Navigating the Dementia Journey
Chapter 4: Managing the Early Stages

- Non-Verbal Communication: Using gestures, facial expressions, and touch can enhance communication, especially when verbal skills decline.

Creating a Supportive Environment

A safe and familiar environment can reduce anxiety and confusion.

- Home Modifications: Making necessary adjustments to the home, such as removing tripping hazards and installing safety features, can enhance independence and safety.

- Routine Establishment: Consistent daily routines provide a sense of structure and reduce uncertainty.

- Social Engagement: Encouraging participation in social activities and maintaining connections with friends and family can help prevent isolation.

Part II: Navigating the Dementia Journey
Chapter 4: Managing the Early Stages

Caregiver Self-Care

- Caring for someone with dementia can be demanding. It's essential for caregivers to prioritize their own well-being.

- Respite Care: Utilizing respite care services allows caregivers to rest and recharge.

- Support Groups: Connecting with other caregivers can provide emotional support and practical advice.

- Self-Care Activities: Engaging in hobbies, exercise, and relaxation techniques can help manage stress.

By implementing these strategies, caregivers can create a supportive environment that promotes the well-being of the person with dementia while also caring for themselves.

Part II: Navigating the Dementia Journey
Chapter 5: Understanding Brain Disorders

Brain disorders form a complex web of conditions that can significantly impact cognitive function. Let's delve into some of the key brain disorders linked to dementia.

Alzheimer's Disease

- Often considered the most common form of dementia, Alzheimer's disease is a progressive neurodegenerative disorder that gradually destroys memory and thinking skills. It's characterized by the formation of abnormal protein clumps in the brain called amyloid plaques and tau tangles.

Vascular Dementia
- Caused by reduced blood flow to the brain, vascular dementia can occur after a stroke or due to chronic conditions like high blood pressure or diabetes. Symptoms can vary widely depending on the areas of the brain affected.

Lewy Body Dementia

- In this condition, abnormal protein deposits called Lewy bodies build up in the brain, affecting thinking, movement, and behavior. People with Lewy body dementia often experience visual hallucinations and sleep disturbances.

Part II: Navigating the Dementia Journey
Chapter 5: Understanding Brain Disorders

Frontotemporal Dementia

- Primarily affecting the frontal and temporal lobes of the brain, frontotemporal dementia leads to changes in personality, behavior, and language. It often develops earlier in life compared to other types of dementia.

Mixed Dementia

- Many individuals with dementia have a combination of different brain disorders, such as Alzheimer's and vascular dementia. This is known as mixed dementia.

- It's crucial to note that while these are some of the most common brain disorders linked to dementia, there are many other conditions that can contribute to cognitive decline.

Part II: Navigating the Dementia Journey
Chapter 5: Understanding Brain Disorders
5.1- Alcohol and Dementia

Alcohol consumption and dementia have a complex relationship. While moderate alcohol consumption has not been definitively linked to an increased risk of dementia, excessive and prolonged alcohol use can lead to serious brain damage.

Alcohol-Related Brain Injury (ARBI)

ARBI is the term now used instead of "alcohol-related dementia." It encompasses the range of cognitive impairments caused by excessive alcohol consumption over a prolonged period.

Symptoms of ARBI can include:

- Memory problems
- Difficulty concentrating
- Problems with decision-making
- Personality changes
- Mood swings
- Physical symptoms like tremors, unsteady gait, and eye problems

Part II: Navigating the Dementia Journey
Chapter 5: Understanding Brain Disorders
5.1- Alcohol and Dementia

How Alcohol Damages the Brain

Excessive alcohol consumption can lead to:

- Brain cell damage: Alcohol directly harms brain cells, leading to cognitive decline.

- Nutritional deficiencies: Alcohol can interfere with the absorption of essential nutrients, further impacting brain health.

- Increased risk of accidents: Alcohol-related accidents can cause brain injuries.

Prevention and Treatment

- The best way to prevent ARBI is to avoid excessive alcohol consumption. If you or someone you know has concerns about alcohol use and its impact on brain health, it's essential to seek professional help. Treatment often involves alcohol detoxification, counseling, and support groups.

- It's important to note that while alcohol abuse can significantly increase the risk of dementia, it's not the only factor. Other lifestyle factors, such as diet, exercise, and mental stimulation, also play crucial roles in brain health.

Part II: Navigating the Dementia Journey
Chapter 5: Understanding Brain Disorders
5.2- Alzheimer's Disease

Alzheimer's disease is the most common form of dementia, a progressive brain disorder that gradually erodes memory and thinking skills. It's a complex disease with a significant impact on individuals, families, and society.

Understanding the Disease

- Brain Changes: Alzheimer's is characterized by the buildup of abnormal proteins in the brain: amyloid plaques and tau tangles. These disrupt communication between brain cells, leading to their eventual death.

- Progressive Nature: The disease progresses gradually, with symptoms worsening over time. Early stages may involve mild memory loss, while later stages can lead to severe cognitive decline and difficulty with basic tasks.

- Risk Factors: While the exact causes of Alzheimer's are unknown, several factors increase the risk, including age, family history, and certain genetic mutations.

Part II: Navigating the Dementia Journey
Chapter 5: Understanding Brain Disorders
5.2- Alzheimer's Disease

Symptoms of Alzheimer's

Symptoms can vary from person to person and progress at different rates. Common signs include:

- Memory loss: Difficulty remembering recent events, names, or appointments.

- Challenges with thinking and problem-solving: Trouble with planning, organizing, and completing familiar tasks.

- Language difficulties: Finding the right words, following conversations, or reading.

- Changes in mood and behavior: Increased irritability, agitation, or apathy.

- Visual spatial challenges: Difficulty with depth perception, judging distances, and recognizing objects.

Part II: Navigating the Dementia Journey
Chapter 5: Understanding Brain Disorders
5.2- Alzheimer's Disease

Current Research and Treatment

While there's no cure for Alzheimer's, research is ongoing to develop effective treatments and prevention strategies. Current treatments focus on managing symptoms and slowing disease progression.

- Medications: Available drugs can help manage some symptoms of Alzheimer's, but they don't stop the disease.

- Lifestyle factors: Maintaining a healthy lifestyle, including regular exercise, a balanced diet, and cognitive stimulation, can support brain health.

- Support and care: Providing a supportive environment and understanding the challenges faced by individuals with Alzheimer's is crucial.

Would you like to explore specific aspects of Alzheimer's disease, such as its impact on caregivers, the latest research developments, or strategies for coping with the disease?

Part II: Navigating the Dementia Journey
Chapter 5: Understanding Brain Disorders
5.3- Amnestic Mild Cognitive Impairment

Amnestic Mild Cognitive Impairment (aMCI) is a stage between normal aging and dementia. It primarily affects memory, with individuals experiencing more significant memory problems than typically expected for their age. However, these memory issues do not yet severely interfere with daily life activities.

Key Characteristics of aMCI

- Memory loss: This is the primary symptom. People with aMCI may forget important information, appointments, or conversations.

- Preserved daily living skills: Unlike dementia, individuals with aMCI can generally manage daily tasks independently.

- Increased risk for Alzheimer's disease: People with aMCI are at a higher risk of developing Alzheimer's disease compared to the general population.

Part II: Navigating the Dementia Journey
Chapter 5: Understanding Brain Disorders
5.3- Amnestic Mild Cognitive Impairment

Differentiating aMCI from Normal Aging

It's essential to distinguish between normal age-related memory lapses and aMCI. While forgetting minor details occasionally is normal, persistent and significant memory problems that impact daily life may indicate aMCI.

Diagnosis and Management

Diagnosing aMCI involves a comprehensive evaluation, including medical history, cognitive tests, and brain imaging. Early detection is crucial as it allows for monitoring and potential interventions to slow cognitive decline. Management of aMCI focuses on:

- Lifestyle modifications: Regular exercise, a healthy diet, and mental stimulation can help improve cognitive function.

- Medication: Some medications may be prescribed to address specific symptoms, such as sleep disturbances or mood changes.

- Support and monitoring: Regular check-ups and involvement in support groups can provide emotional support and information about the condition.

It's important to note that while aMCI is a serious condition, not everyone with aMCI will develop Alzheimer's disease. Many individuals with aMCI maintain a good quality of life for several years.

Part II: Navigating the Dementia Journey
Chapter 5: Understanding Brain Disorders
5.4- Cerebral Amyloid Angiopathy

Cerebral Amyloid Angiopathy (CAA) is a condition where amyloid proteins build up in the walls of the brain's blood vessels. This buildup weakens the blood vessels, making them more prone to bleeding.

Key Characteristics of CAA

- Amyloid buildup: The accumulation of amyloid protein in the blood vessels is the primary feature.

- Hemorrhage: The weakened blood vessels can rupture, leading to bleeding in the brain, which is often referred to as lobar hemorrhage.

- Cognitive decline: In some cases, CAA can contribute to cognitive decline, although this is less common than in other types of dementia.

Symptoms of CAA

Symptoms can vary depending on the severity and location of the bleeding. They may include:

- Sudden, severe headache: Often associated with a hemorrhage.
- Weakness or numbness: Particularly on one side of the body.
- Difficulty speaking or understanding speech.
- Vision problems.
- Seizures.

Part II: Navigating the Dementia Journey
Chapter 5: Understanding Brain Disorders
5.4- Cerebral Amyloid Angiopathy

- Cognitive changes: In some cases, memory problems and other cognitive difficulties may occur.

Risk Factors

- Age: The risk increases with age.
- Genetics: A family history of CAA or Alzheimer's disease can increase the risk.
- Down syndrome: Individuals with Down syndrome have a higher risk of developing CAA.

Diagnosis and Treatment

- Diagnosing CAA can be challenging as symptoms may overlap with other conditions. Imaging tests, such as MRI or CT scans, can help identify bleeding in the brain.

- Treatment focuses on managing symptoms and preventing further bleeding. Medications to control blood pressure and prevent blood clots may be prescribed. In cases of severe bleeding, surgical intervention may be necessary.

Part II: Navigating the Dementia Journey
Chapter 5: Understanding Brain Disorders
5.5- Neuroplasticity and Dementia

Neuroplasticity is the brain's ability to reorganize itself by forming new neural connections throughout life. It allows the brain to adapt to new experiences, learn, and form new memories.

While neuroplasticity is a remarkable property of the brain, its role in dementia is complex.

Neuroplasticity in the Context of Dementia

- Decline in Neuroplasticity: In dementia, the brain's ability to form new connections diminishes, contributing to cognitive decline.

- Compensatory Mechanisms: The brain may attempt to compensate for damaged areas by creating new neural pathways. However, this compensatory capacity is often limited in dementia.

- Potential for Intervention: Understanding neuroplasticity has led to the exploration of strategies to stimulate brain activity and potentially slow cognitive decline.

Part II: Navigating the Dementia Journey
Chapter 5: Understanding Brain Disorders
5.5- Neuroplasticity and Dementia

Harnessing Neuroplasticity for Dementia Care

While research is ongoing, some approaches that aim to stimulate neuroplasticity include:

- Cognitive stimulation: Engaging in mentally challenging activities like puzzles, games, and learning new skills.

- Physical exercise: Regular physical activity has been linked to improved brain health and cognitive function.

- Social interaction: Maintaining social connections can stimulate the brain and provide emotional support.

- Music and art therapy: These activities can engage different areas of the brain and promote creativity.

It's essential to note that while these approaches may help to slow cognitive decline and improve quality of life, they are not a cure for dementia.

Part II: Navigating the Dementia Journey
Chapter 5: Understanding Brain Disorders
5.6- Neurotransmitters and Dementia

Neurotransmitters are chemical messengers that transmit signals between nerve cells. They play a crucial role in various brain functions, including memory, mood, and movement. In dementia, the balance of these neurotransmitters is often disrupted.

Key Neurotransmitters Involved in Dementia

- Acetylcholine: This neurotransmitter is essential for memory and learning. Its levels decline significantly in Alzheimer's disease.

- Dopamine: Involved in movement, motivation, and reward, dopamine levels are affected in conditions like Parkinson's disease and dementia with Lewy bodies.

- Noradrenaline (norepinephrine): This neurotransmitter plays a role in attention, arousal, and mood. It's associated with conditions like Alzheimer's and vascular dementia.

- Serotonin: Linked to mood, sleep, appetite, and pain, serotonin imbalances can contribute to depression, anxiety, and sleep disturbances common in dementia.

- Glutamate: As the primary excitatory neurotransmitter, glutamate is involved in learning and memory. However, excessive glutamate levels can be toxic to neurons, contributing to neuronal death in conditions like Alzheimer's disease.

Part II: Navigating the Dementia Journey
Chapter 5: Understanding Brain Disorders
5.6- Neurotransmitters and Dementia

The Role of Neurotransmitters in Dementia

- Communication Breakdown: The decline in neurotransmitters disrupts communication between brain cells, leading to cognitive impairment.

- Symptom Manifestation: Changes in neurotransmitter levels contribute to the various symptoms of dementia, such as memory loss, mood changes, and movement difficulties.

- Therapeutic Targets: Understanding the role of neurotransmitters has led to the development of medications that target specific neurotransmitter systems.

While research continues to unravel the complex interplay between neurotransmitters and dementia, it's clear that these chemical messengers play a vital role in the progression of the disease.

Part II: Navigating the Dementia Journey
Chapter 5: Understanding Brain Disorders
5.7- Electrical Signaling and Dementia

The human brain is a complex network of billions of neurons that communicate through electrical and chemical signals. In a healthy brain, this communication is precise and efficient, allowing for complex cognitive functions. However, in dementia, this intricate system is disrupted.

The Role of Electrical Signals in Brain Function

- Neuron Firing: Neurons communicate by sending electrical impulses, known as action potentials, along their axons.

- Synaptic Transmission: When an electrical signal reaches the end of an axon, it triggers the release of neurotransmitters, which bind to receptors on neighboring neurons, initiating a new electrical signal.

- Neural Networks: The brain operates through complex networks of interconnected neurons. Efficient electrical signaling is crucial for information processing and memory formation.

Part II: Navigating the Dementia Journey
Chapter 5: Understanding Brain Disorders
5.7- Electrical Signaling and Dementia

Electrical Signaling in Dementia

In dementia, the electrical activity of the brain is impaired. This can manifest in several ways:

- Reduced neuronal firing: Brain cells may become less active, leading to slower processing speed and cognitive decline.

- Abnormal brain rhythms: The synchronized electrical activity of brain cells, known as brainwaves, can become irregular in dementia.

- Synaptic dysfunction: The connections between neurons weaken, affecting communication and memory formation.

Part II: Navigating the Dementia Journey
Chapter 5: Understanding Brain Disorders
5.7- Electrical Signaling and Dementia

Research and Potential Implications

Understanding the changes in electrical signaling in dementia is crucial for developing new treatments and diagnostic tools. Some potential applications include:

- Early detection: Identifying abnormal brain electrical patterns could aid in early diagnosis.

- Disease progression monitoring: Tracking changes in brain electrical activity can help monitor disease progression.

- Therapeutic interventions: Developing techniques to modulate brain electrical activity, such as deep brain stimulation, may offer potential treatment options.

While research is still in its early stages, the study of electrical signaling in dementia holds promise for improving the lives of those affected by this devastating condition.

Part II: Navigating the Dementia Journey
Chapter 6: Medical Care and Management

The Evaluation of the Person with Dementia

A comprehensive evaluation is essential for developing an effective care plan for someone with dementia. This involves a thorough assessment of the individual's cognitive, physical, and emotional state.

- Cognitive Assessment: Evaluating memory, attention, language, and problem-solving skills to determine the stage of dementia.

- Physical Examination: Checking for underlying medical conditions that may contribute to cognitive decline or worsen symptoms.

- Functional Assessment: Assessing daily living activities to identify areas where assistance may be needed.

- Behavioral Assessment: Observing and documenting any behavioral changes or challenges.

- Caregiver Interview: Gathering information about the person's history, symptoms, and the impact of dementia on the caregiver.

Part II: Navigating the Dementia Journey
Chapter 6: Medical Care and Management

Medical Treatment and Management of Dementia

While there's no cure for dementia, medical interventions can help manage symptoms and improve quality of life.

- Medications: Certain medications may be prescribed to address specific symptoms, such as memory loss, agitation, or sleep disturbances.

- Regular Check-ups: Regular medical evaluations are crucial to monitor the progression of dementia and address any new health issues.

- Disease-Modifying Therapies: Ongoing research is exploring potential treatments to slow or halt the progression of dementia.

Part II: Navigating the Dementia Journey
Chapter 6: Medical Care and Management

Common Medical Problems in Dementia

Individuals with dementia are at increased risk for various medical complications.

- Pain Management: Identifying and treating pain effectively is essential for comfort and quality of life.

- Dehydration: Monitoring fluid intake and addressing swallowing difficulties can help prevent dehydration.

- Pneumonia: Implementing preventive measures, such as vaccination and good oral hygiene, can reduce the risk of pneumonia.

- Constipation: Dietary adjustments, increased fluid intake, and exercise can help alleviate constipation.

- Vision Problems: Regular eye exams and appropriate vision aids can improve quality of life.

- Nutrition: Ensuring adequate nutrition is crucial for overall health.

Part II: Navigating the Dementia Journey
Chapter 6: Medical Care and Management
6.1- Evaluating the Person with Dementia

A comprehensive evaluation is essential for understanding the specific needs and challenges faced by an individual with dementia. This process involves gathering information from multiple sources, including the person with dementia, their caregivers, and healthcare professionals.

Key Components of a Dementia Evaluation

1. Cognitive Assessment

- Memory evaluation: Assessing short-term and long-term memory, recall, and recognition.

- Attention and concentration: Evaluating the ability to focus and sustain attention.

- Language skills: Assessing comprehension, expression, and naming abilities.

- Visuospatial skills: Evaluating the ability to perceive and manipulate visual information.

- Executive function: Assessing planning, organizing, decision-making, and problem-solving abilities.

Part II: Navigating the Dementia Journey
Chapter 6: Medical Care and Management
6.1- Evaluating the Person with Dementia

Commonly used cognitive assessment tools include:

- Mini-Mental State Examination (MMSE)
- Montreal Cognitive Assessment (MoCA)
- Clock Drawing Test

2. Functional Assessment

- Activities of daily living (ADLs): Evaluating the ability to perform basic self-care tasks like bathing, dressing, and eating.

- Instrumental activities of daily living (IADLs): Assessing the ability to manage household tasks, finances, and transportation.

- Behavioral assessment: Observing and documenting any behavioral changes or challenges, such as agitation, wandering, or sleep disturbances.

3. Physical Examination

- General health assessment: Identifying any underlying medical conditions that could contribute to cognitive decline.

- Neurological examination: Assessing motor skills, reflexes, and sensory functions.

- Sensory evaluation: Checking vision, hearing, and touch to rule out sensory impairments that might affect cognitive function.

Part II: Navigating the Dementia Journey
Chapter 6: Medical Care and Management
6.1- Evaluating the Person with Dementia

4. Caregiver Interview

- Caregiver burden: Assessing the impact of caregiving on the caregiver's physical and emotional well-being.

- Caregiver needs: Identifying the caregiver's support needs and providing resources.

- Caregiver coping strategies: Exploring the caregiver's coping mechanisms and offering support.

Importance of a Comprehensive Evaluation
A thorough evaluation provides a baseline for developing a personalized care plan. It helps identify strengths and weaknesses, determine the stage of dementia, and address specific needs. Regular re-evaluations are essential to monitor changes in cognitive function and adjust the care plan accordingly.

Part II: Navigating the Dementia Journey
Chapter 6: Medical Care and Management
6.2- Medical Treatment and Management

While there's no cure for dementia, medical interventions can significantly improve quality of life for individuals with the condition and their caregivers. Treatment focuses on managing symptoms, slowing disease progression, and addressing related health issues.

Medications for Dementia

Several types of medications are used to manage dementia symptoms:

- Cholinesterase inhibitors: These drugs help improve cognitive function by increasing levels of acetylcholine, a neurotransmitter important for memory. Examples include donepezil, rivastigmine, and galantamine.

- Memantine: This medication regulates the activity of the neurotransmitter glutamate, which can be excessive in the brains of people with Alzheimer's disease.

- Other medications: Depending on specific symptoms, antidepressants, antipsychotics, or mood stabilizers may be prescribed.

Part II: Navigating the Dementia Journey
Chapter 6: Medical Care and Management
6.2- Medical Treatment and Management

It's essential to note that medications are not a cure for dementia but can help manage symptoms temporarily.

Importance of Regular Check-ups

Regular medical evaluations are crucial for monitoring the progression of dementia, identifying potential complications, and adjusting treatment plans as needed. These check-ups involve:

- Cognitive assessments: To track changes in cognitive function.

- Physical examinations: To monitor overall health and identify any new medical conditions.

- Medication reviews: To ensure medications are effective and safe.

- Caregiver support: Providing guidance and resources for caregivers.

Part II: Navigating the Dementia Journey
Chapter 6: Medical Care and Management
6.2- Medical Treatment and Management

Managing Comorbidities

Individuals with dementia often have other health conditions, which can complicate care. It's essential to address these comorbidities to improve overall well-being. Common comorbidities include:

- Heart disease: Managing blood pressure, cholesterol, and diabetes.

- Diabetes: Monitoring blood sugar levels and preventing complications.

- Urinary incontinence: Implementing bladder training and incontinence products.

- Sleep disturbances: Addressing sleep problems through sleep hygiene and medication if necessary.

Advance Care Planning

As dementia progresses, it's important to have open conversations about end-of-life care and create advance directives. This involves discussing treatment preferences and appointing a healthcare power of attorney.

Part II: Navigating the Dementia Journey
Chapter 6: Medical Care and Management
6.3- Common Medical Challenges (pain, dehydration, pneumonia, constipation, vision problems, etc.)

Individuals with dementia often experience a range of medical challenges that can significantly impact their quality of life.

- **Pain** is a common issue that can be difficult to identify and manage in people with dementia. They may struggle to communicate their discomfort, leading to increased frustration and agitation. It's essential to observe for nonverbal signs of pain, such as facial expressions, restlessness, or changes in behavior.

- **Dehydration** is another concern due to factors like decreased thirst sensation, difficulty swallowing, or simply forgetting to drink. Monitoring fluid intake and encouraging regular hydration is crucial.

- **Pneumonia** is a serious risk for people with dementia due to weakened immune systems and difficulty clearing secretions. Regular vaccinations and preventative measures like good oral hygiene can help reduce the risk.

- **Constipation** is a common digestive issue that can be uncomfortable and contribute to other problems. Increasing fiber intake, staying hydrated, and regular exercise can help alleviate constipation.

Part II: Navigating the Dementia Journey
Chapter 6: Medical Care and Management
6.3- Common Medical Challenges (pain, dehydration, pneumonia, constipation, vision problems, etc.)

- **Vision problems** can significantly impact daily life for individuals with dementia. Regular eye exams and appropriate vision aids can improve their quality of life and safety.

These are just some of the common medical challenges associated with dementia. It's important to remember that each person's experience is unique, and careful monitoring and management are essential for optimal care.

Part II: Navigating the Dementia Journey
Chapter 6: Medical Care and Management
6.3- Common Medical Challenges (pain, dehydration, pneumonia, constipation, vision problems, etc.)

In addition to the challenges we've already discussed, individuals with dementia often face other medical issues that can significantly impact their quality of life.

Neurological Issues
- Seizures: While uncommon, seizures can occur in some types of dementia.
- Sleep disturbances: Sleep problems, such as insomnia or excessive daytime sleepiness, are common and can contribute to agitation and behavioral changes.
- Motor difficulties: As dementia progresses, individuals may experience difficulties with balance, coordination, and mobility.

Mental Health Challenges
- Depression: Depression is common among people with dementia and can worsen cognitive symptoms.
- Anxiety: Anxiety can manifest as agitation, restlessness, or fearfulness.
- Psychosis: In some cases, individuals with dementia may experience delusions or hallucinations.

Nutritional Challenges
- Weight loss: Unintentional weight loss can occur due to decreased appetite, difficulty swallowing, or changes in taste.
- Malnutrition: Inadequate nutrition can lead to a decline in overall health and well-being.

Part II: Navigating the Dementia Journey
Chapter 6: Medical Care and Management
6.3- Common Medical Challenges (pain, dehydration, pneumonia, constipation, vision problems, etc.)

Skin Issues

- Pressure ulcers: Due to immobility, individuals with dementia are at increased risk of developing pressure ulcers.
- Urinary and fecal incontinence: These issues can lead to skin breakdown and infections.

It's important to note that these are just some of the additional medical challenges that can arise in people with dementia. Early identification and management of these issues can help improve quality of life and prevent complications.

Part II: Navigating the Dementia Journey
Chapter 7: Prevention and Symptom Management
7.1- Preventing Dementia

While there's no guaranteed way to prevent dementia, research suggests that adopting a healthy lifestyle can significantly reduce the risk.

Key Lifestyle Factors for Dementia Prevention

- **Heart Health:**
    - Manage blood pressure: High blood pressure is a significant risk factor.
    - Control cholesterol: High cholesterol can contribute to heart disease and stroke, both linked to dementia.
    - Maintain a healthy weight: Obesity is associated with an increased risk of dementia.
    - Regular exercise: Physical activity benefits both heart and brain health.

- **Diet:**
    - Mediterranean diet: Rich in fruits, vegetables, whole grains, and healthy fats, this diet has shown promise in reducing dementia risk.
    - Limit processed foods: High intake of processed foods is linked to increased risk.

- **Mental Stimulation:**
    - Lifelong learning: Engage in activities that challenge your mind, such as puzzles, reading, or learning new skills.
    - Social interaction: Maintain strong social connections.

Part II: Navigating the Dementia Journey
Chapter 7: Prevention and Symptom Management
7.1- Preventing Dementia

- **Physical Activity:**
  - Regular exercise improves brain health and reduces the risk of chronic diseases.

- **Sleep:**
  - Prioritize quality sleep for optimal brain function.

- **Avoid Harmful Substances:**
  - Refrain from smoking and excessive alcohol consumption.

- **Manage Stress:**
  - Chronic stress can negatively impact brain health. Find healthy ways to manage stress.

Early Detection and Intervention

Even if dementia cannot be entirely prevented, early detection and intervention can significantly improve quality of life. Regular check-ups, especially after the age of 65, can help identify early signs of cognitive decline.

Part II: Navigating the Dementia Journey
Chapter 7: Prevention and Symptom Management
7.2- Decreasing Dementia Symptoms

While there's no cure for dementia, various strategies can help manage symptoms and improve quality of life for individuals with the condition.

Lifestyle Modifications

- Physical Activity: Regular exercise has been shown to improve cognitive function and mood.

- Mental Stimulation: Engaging in mentally stimulating activities like puzzles, games, or learning new skills can help maintain cognitive abilities.

- Social Interaction: Maintaining social connections can reduce feelings of isolation and loneliness, which can contribute to cognitive decline.

- Healthy Diet: A balanced diet rich in fruits, vegetables, whole grains, and lean protein can support overall health and brain function.

- Adequate Sleep: Ensuring sufficient sleep is crucial for cognitive function and overall well-being.

Part II: Navigating the Dementia Journey
Chapter 7: Prevention and Symptom Management
7.2- Decreasing Dementia Symptoms

Medication

Medication can help manage certain symptoms of dementia, such as memory loss, agitation, and sleep disturbances. It's essential to work closely with a healthcare provider to determine the most appropriate treatment plan.

Environmental Adaptations

Creating a safe and supportive environment can significantly improve the quality of life for individuals with dementia.

- Home safety: Remove hazards and install safety features like grab bars.

- Routine establishment: Consistent daily routines can help reduce confusion and anxiety.

- Visual cues: Using clear and simple visual cues can aid in orientation and communication.

Caregiver Support

Caregivers play a vital role in managing dementia symptoms. Support groups, respite care, and education can help caregivers cope with the challenges of caregiving.

Part II: Navigating the Dementia Journey
Chapter 7: Prevention and Symptom Management
7.3- Managing Memory Problems

Memory loss is a hallmark symptom of dementia, but there are strategies to help manage its impact. Here are some effective approaches:

Environmental Strategies
- Create a memory-friendly environment: Reduce distractions, use clear signage, and maintain consistent routines.
- Utilize memory aids: Calendars, planners, and digital reminders can be helpful tools.
- Label belongings: Labeling items can aid in identification and retrieval.

Communication Techniques
- Simplify language: Use clear and concise language, avoiding complex sentences.
- Provide cues: Offer visual or verbal cues to help with recall.
- Be patient and supportive: Avoid frustration or criticism, which can increase anxiety.

Daily Living Tips
- Maintain routines: Consistent daily routines can help orient individuals with dementia.
- Break tasks into smaller steps: Simplify complex tasks to make them more manageable.
- Use visual aids: Pictures or diagrams can be helpful for explaining tasks or conveying information.

Part II: Navigating the Dementia Journey
Chapter 7: Prevention and Symptom Management
7.3- Managing Memory Problems

Safety Considerations
- Supervision: Provide necessary supervision to prevent accidents and injuries.
- Secure valuables: Keep important items, such as medications and financial documents, in a safe place.

Professional Support
- Consult with a healthcare provider: Discuss available treatment options and explore strategies for managing memory loss.
- Seek support groups: Connecting with other caregivers can provide valuable insights and emotional support.

It's important to remember that while memory loss is a challenging aspect of dementia, with the right strategies and support, it's possible to maintain a good quality of life.

Part III: Caring for the Caregiver
Chapter 8: Prioritizing Self-Care

Caregiving for someone with dementia is demanding and can take an emotional and physical toll. Prioritizing self-care is essential for maintaining your own well-being and ability to provide effective care.

Understanding the Importance of Self-Care

- Preventing burnout: Self-care helps to prevent caregiver burnout, which can lead to physical and emotional exhaustion.

- Improving mood: Taking time for yourself can boost your mood and reduce stress levels.

- Enhancing patience: Self-care can help you maintain patience and empathy in your caregiving role.

- Strengthening relationships: Spending time on yourself can help you maintain strong relationships with family and friends.

Part III: Caring for the Caregiver
Chapter 8: Prioritizing Self-Care

Practical Self-Care Strategies

- **Physical well-being:**
  - Regular exercise: Even short bursts of physical activity can make a difference.
  - Healthy diet: Nourishing your body with balanced meals is crucial.
  - Sufficient sleep: Prioritize quality sleep to recharge your energy.

- **Emotional well-being:**
  - Mindfulness and meditation: These practices can help reduce stress and improve focus.
  - Hobbies and interests: Engaging in activities you enjoy can provide a much-needed escape.
  - Support networks: Connect with friends, family, or support groups for emotional support.

- **Practical support:**
  - Respite care: Utilize respite services to give yourself a break.
  - Time management: Learn to prioritize tasks and delegate when possible.
  - Setting boundaries: It's okay to say no to additional responsibilities.

Remember, self-care is not selfish; it's essential for your ability to provide the best possible care for your loved one.

Part III: Caring for the Caregiver
Chapter 8: Prioritizing Self-Care
8.1- The Impact of Caregiving

Caregiving for a loved one with dementia is a demanding role that can significantly impact a caregiver's physical, emotional, and mental well-being.

Physical Impact

- Chronic stress: The constant demands of caregiving can lead to elevated stress levels, which can weaken the immune system and contribute to various health problems.

- Sleep disturbances: Irregular sleep patterns, due to nighttime caregiving responsibilities or worry, can affect overall health.

- Neglect of self-care: Caregivers often prioritize the needs of the person with dementia over their own, leading to poor nutrition, lack of exercise, and inadequate rest.

- Increased risk of illness: Due to weakened immune systems, caregivers are more susceptible to infections.

Part III: Caring for the Caregiver
Chapter 8: Prioritizing Self-Care
8.1- The Impact of Caregiving

Emotional Impact

- Depression: The constant challenges of caregiving can lead to feelings of sadness, hopelessness, and isolation.

- Anxiety: Worrying about the person with dementia's well-being can contribute to anxiety and stress.

- Guilt: Caregivers may experience guilt for feeling overwhelmed or resentful.

- Grief: As the disease progresses, caregivers may experience anticipatory grief and loss.

Social Impact

- Isolation: Caregiving responsibilities can limit social interactions and lead to feelings of isolation.

- Strained relationships: The demands of caregiving can put a strain on relationships with family and friends.

- Financial strain: Caregiving can be financially burdensome, leading to stress and anxiety.

Understanding the impact of caregiving is crucial for seeking support and implementing strategies to maintain well-being.

Part III: Caring for the Caregiver
Chapter 8: Prioritizing Self-Care
8.2- Caregiver Burnout

Caregiver burnout is a serious issue that can significantly impact your physical, emotional, and mental health. It's essential to recognize the signs of burnout to take steps to prevent or manage it.

Symptoms of Caregiver Burnout

- Physical symptoms: Fatigue, frequent illness, changes in appetite, sleep disturbances.
- Emotional symptoms: Feeling overwhelmed, irritable, depressed, or anxious.
- Behavioral symptoms: Neglecting personal needs, withdrawing from social activities, increased use of alcohol or drugs.
- Cognitive symptoms: Difficulty concentrating, forgetfulness, and indecision.

Impact of Caregiver Burnout

Burnout can have far-reaching consequences, including:
- Increased risk of health problems: Physical and mental health issues can worsen.
- Strained relationships: Burnout can impact relationships with family, friends, and the person being cared for.
- Reduced quality of care: When caregivers are overwhelmed, the quality of care provided may decline.

It's important to remember that experiencing some of these symptoms doesn't necessarily mean you have burnout, but it's a sign to pay attention to your well-being.

Part III: Caring for the Caregiver
Chapter 8: Prioritizing Self-Care
8.3- Preparing for the Caregiving Journey

Preparing for the caregiving journey can be overwhelming, but it's essential to lay a solid foundation for providing effective care. Here are some key steps:

Education and Information
- Understand the condition: Learn about dementia, its progression, and available treatment options.
- Seek professional advice: Consult with doctors, nurses, and social workers for guidance.
- Attend support groups: Connect with other caregivers to share experiences and learn coping strategies.

Legal and Financial Planning
- Power of attorney: Appoint someone to make financial and healthcare decisions on behalf of the person with dementia.
- Advance directives: Create documents outlining the person's wishes for medical care in case they are unable to communicate.
- Financial planning: Assess financial resources and explore potential funding options, such as long-term care insurance.
- Estate planning: Consider creating a will or trust to ensure the person's assets are managed according to their wishes.

Part III: Caring for the Caregiver
Chapter 8: Prioritizing Self-Care
8.3- Preparing for the Caregiving Journey

Home Safety and Modifications

- Assess the home: Identify potential hazards and make necessary adjustments.
- Install safety equipment: Consider installing grab bars, ramps, and other safety features.
- Create a safe environment: Remove tripping hazards and clutter to prevent accidents.

Building a Support Network

- Involve family and friends: Enlist their help with caregiving tasks or emotional support.
- Seek professional help: Consider hiring home health aides or other care providers.
- Join support groups: Connect with other caregivers for shared experiences and advice.

Self-Care

- Prioritize your well-being: Make time for physical and emotional self-care.
- Set realistic expectations: Understand the limitations of caregiving and avoid overexertion.
- Seek support: Don't hesitate to ask for help when needed.

By taking these steps, you can better prepare for the challenges of caregiving and provide the best possible care for your loved one.

Part III: Caring for the Caregiver
Chapter 8: Prioritizing Self-Care
8.4- Maintaining Physical and Mental Health

Caring for someone with dementia can be physically and emotionally demanding. Prioritizing your own health is essential for your ability to provide effective care.

Physical Health
- Regular exercise: Aim for at least 30 minutes of moderate-intensity exercise most days of the week. Even short bursts of activity can make a difference.
- Healthy diet: Focus on nutrient-rich foods like fruits, vegetables, whole grains, and lean proteins.
- Adequate sleep: Prioritize quality sleep by creating a relaxing bedtime routine and ensuring a comfortable sleep environment.
- Regular check-ups: Schedule regular medical appointments to monitor your overall health.

Mental Health
- Stress management: Practice relaxation techniques like deep breathing, meditation, or yoga.
- Emotional expression: Talk to friends, family, or a therapist about your feelings.
- Social connection: Maintain social relationships and engage in activities you enjoy.
- Time for yourself: Schedule breaks and hobbies to recharge.
- Seek professional help: Don't hesitate to consult a mental health professional if you're struggling.

Part III: Caring for the Caregiver
Chapter 8: Prioritizing Self-Care
8.4- Maintaining Physical and Mental Health

Balancing Caregiving and Self-Care

- Time management: Prioritize tasks and delegate when possible.
- Respite care: Utilize respite services to give yourself a break.
- Setting boundaries: Learn to say no and establish boundaries to protect your time and energy.

Remember, taking care of yourself is not selfish; it's essential for your ability to provide effective care for your loved one.

Part III: Caring for the Caregiver
Chapter 8: Prioritizing Self-Care
8.5- Building Resilience

Resilience is the ability to bounce back from adversity. For caregivers, building resilience is essential for coping with the challenges of dementia care.

Strategies for Building Resilience
- Mindfulness and Meditation: These practices can help you focus on the present moment, reducing stress and anxiety.
- Support Networks: Connect with other caregivers, family, or friends for emotional support and practical assistance.
- Healthy Lifestyle: Prioritize physical activity, a balanced diet, and sufficient sleep.
- Setting Boundaries: Learn to say no and establish boundaries to protect your time and energy.
- Positive Thinking: Focus on the positive aspects of your caregiving role and find gratitude in small moments.
- Learning and Growth: Seek opportunities for personal growth and development.
- Self-Compassion: Be kind to yourself and avoid self-criticism.

Overcoming Challenges
- Acknowledge your feelings: It's okay to experience a range of emotions.
- Seek professional help: Consider counseling or therapy if needed.
- Take breaks: Utilize respite care or other support services to recharge.
- Celebrate small victories: Recognize your achievements, no matter how small.

Part III: Caring for the Caregiver
Chapter 8: Prioritizing Self-Care
8.5- Building Resilience

Remember, building resilience is an ongoing process. It's important to be patient with yourself and allow time for growth and adaptation.

Part III: Caring for the Caregiver
Chapter 8: Prioritizing Self-Care
8.6- Managing Emotional Reactions

Caregiving can evoke a wide range of emotions, from sadness and frustration to anger and guilt. It's essential to develop strategies for managing these emotions to maintain your well-being.

Understanding Your Emotions
- Acknowledge your feelings: It's important to recognize and validate your emotions without judgment.
- Identify triggers: Understanding what situations or behaviors trigger specific emotions can help you develop coping strategies.
- Practice self-compassion: Be kind to yourself and avoid self-blame.

Coping Strategies
- Communication: Talk to trusted friends, family, or a therapist about your feelings.
- Stress management techniques: Incorporate relaxation techniques like deep breathing, meditation, or yoga into your routine.
- Time management: Prioritize tasks and schedule breaks to prevent feeling overwhelmed.
- Setting boundaries: Learn to say no and establish limits to protect your emotional well-being.
- Seek support: Join a support group or connect with other caregivers to share experiences and advice.

Part III: Caring for the Caregiver
Chapter 8: Prioritizing Self-Care
8.6- Managing Emotional Reactions

Managing Difficult Behaviors
- Remain calm: Respond to challenging behaviors with patience and understanding.
- Avoid confrontation: Try to de-escalate situations through redirection or distraction.
- Seek professional help: Consult with a healthcare provider or dementia specialist for guidance.

Remember, it's okay to feel a range of emotions as a caregiver. By developing effective coping strategies, you can better manage your emotional well-being and provide the best possible care for your loved one.

Dealing with Challenging Behaviors

Challenging behaviors can be one of the most difficult aspects of caregiving. These behaviors can range from agitation and aggression to wandering and resistance to personal care.

Understanding the Cause

- Identify triggers: Try to determine what might be causing the behavior, such as pain, discomfort, or unmet needs.
- Communicate effectively: Use simple, clear language and avoid arguments.
- Create a calm environment: Reduce distractions and maintain a consistent routine.

Part III: Caring for the Caregiver
Chapter 8: Prioritizing Self-Care
8.6- Managing Emotional Reactions

Coping Strategies

- Safety first: Prioritize the safety of both the caregiver and the person with dementia.
- Time management: Break tasks into smaller, manageable steps.
- Respite care: Utilize respite services to give yourself a break.
- Seek professional help: Consult with a healthcare provider or dementia specialist for guidance.
- Join a support group: Connect with other caregivers who understand the challenges.

Self-Care

- Practice self-compassion: Remember that you are doing your best.
- Set boundaries: Establish limits to protect your physical and emotional well-being.
- Seek support: Talk to friends, family, or a therapist about your feelings.

Remember, it's important to approach challenging behaviors with patience and understanding. By implementing these strategies and seeking support, you can better manage these situations and maintain your own well-being.

Part III: Caring for the Caregiver
Chapter 9: Practical Caregiving Strategies

Effective caregiving involves a combination of planning, organization, and practical skills. Here are some strategies to help you navigate the challenges:

Daily Living Activities
- Routine establishment: Consistent daily routines can provide a sense of security for the person with dementia.
- Meal planning: Prepare healthy and easy-to-eat meals. Consider meal delivery services or prepared meals.
- Personal hygiene: Assist with bathing, grooming, and dressing as needed, while encouraging independence.
- Medication management: Use pill organizers or medication reminders to ensure proper adherence.

Home Safety
- Remove hazards: Identify and eliminate potential fall risks, such as loose rugs or clutter.
- Install safety equipment: Consider grab bars, non-slip mats, and adequate lighting.
- Secure exits: Prevent wandering by installing door alarms or locks.

Communication and Engagement
- Simplify language: Use clear and concise language, avoiding complex sentences.
- Use visual aids: Pictures, gestures, and objects can help convey information.
- Encourage social interaction: Engage in activities that promote social connection and stimulation.

Part III: Caring for the Caregiver
Chapter 9: Practical Caregiving Strategies

Managing Challenging Behaviors
- Identify triggers: Try to determine what might be causing the behavior.
- Create a calm environment: Reduce distractions and maintain a consistent routine.
- Redirect attention: Use distractions to divert attention from upsetting situations.
- Seek professional help: Consult with a healthcare provider or dementia specialist for guidance.

Self-Care
- Prioritize your well-being: Schedule time for yourself, even if it's just a few minutes a day.
- Build a support network: Connect with other caregivers for emotional support and practical advice.
- Respite care: Utilize respite services to give yourself a break.

Part III: Caring for the Caregiver
Chapter 9: Practical Caregiving Strategies
9.1- Building Strong Connections

Maintaining strong connections with the person living with dementia is crucial for their well-being. Here are some strategies:

Understanding the Importance of Connection
- Emotional well-being: Strong connections provide a sense of security and belonging.
- Communication: Relationships offer opportunities for meaningful interactions.
- Stimulation: Shared activities can stimulate the mind and prevent isolation.

Building and Maintaining Connections
- Shared activities: Engage in activities that the person enjoys, such as listening to music, looking at photo albums, or going for walks.
- Quality time: Spend one-on-one time focusing on the individual.
- Physical touch: Gentle touch can be comforting and reassuring.
- Affirmation and validation: Reassure the person of your love and support.
- Patience and empathy: Understand that communication and behavior may change.
- Adapt to changes: Be flexible and willing to try new approaches.

Part III: Caring for the Caregiver
Chapter 9: Practical Caregiving Strategies
9.1- Building Strong Connections

Creating a Stimulating Environment
- Familiar surroundings: Maintain a consistent environment to reduce confusion.
- Sensory stimulation: Incorporate visual, auditory, and tactile elements to engage the senses.
- Memory aids: Use photos, calendars, or other visual cues to support memory.

Involving Family and Friends
- Encourage visits: Invite family and friends to spend time with the person with dementia.
- Share memories: Reminiscing together can be a meaningful experience.
- Create a support network: Connect with other caregivers for shared experiences and advice.

Building strong connections requires patience, understanding, and creativity. By focusing on the individual's needs and preferences, you can create a nurturing and supportive environment.

Part III: Caring for the Caregiver
Chapter 9: Practical Caregiving Strategies
9.2- Care Planning and Coordination

A well-structured care plan is essential for managing the complexities of dementia care. It involves coordinating various aspects of care to ensure the person with dementia receives optimal support.

Developing a Comprehensive Care Plan
- Assess needs: Identify the individual's physical, cognitive, and emotional needs.
- Set goals: Establish clear and achievable goals for both the person with dementia and the caregiver.
- Create a schedule: Develop a daily or weekly routine to structure the day.
- Identify resources: Explore available community resources, such as home health aides, adult day care, and support groups.
- Involve the care team: Collaborate with healthcare providers, social workers, and other professionals.

Coordinating Care
- Communication: Maintain open communication with healthcare providers, family members, and other caregivers.
- Information sharing: Share relevant information about the person's condition and care needs.
- Coordination of services: Ensure that different care providers work together seamlessly.
- Regular reviews: Evaluate the care plan regularly and make adjustments as needed.

Part III: Caring for the Caregiver
Chapter 9: Practical Caregiving Strategies
9.2- Care Planning and Coordination

Essential Components of a Care Plan
- Medical care: Include information about medications, doctor appointments, and ongoing health conditions.
- Personal care: Outline daily living activities, such as bathing, dressing, and eating.
- Cognitive support: Include strategies for managing memory loss and cognitive challenges.
- Behavioral management: Address any challenging behaviors and develop coping strategies.
- Safety measures: Identify potential hazards and implement safety precautions.
- Caregiver support: Include plans for respite care, support groups, and self-care.

Tools and Resources
- Care planning software: Consider using digital tools to organize care information.
- Caregiver support groups: Connect with other caregivers for advice and emotional support.
- Local agencies: Explore resources offered by government agencies and community organizations.

Effective care planning and coordination are crucial for providing high-quality care for individuals with dementia. By involving all relevant parties and regularly evaluating the plan, you can ensure the best possible outcomes.

Part III: Caring for the Caregiver
Chapter 9: Practical Caregiving Strategies
9.3- In-Home and Long-Term Care Options

As dementia progresses, the level of care required often increases. Understanding the available options is crucial for making informed decisions.

In-Home Care

In-home care provides assistance with daily living activities while allowing individuals to remain in their familiar surroundings.

- Home health aides: Offer personal care assistance with bathing, dressing, and grooming.
- Homemakers: Provide household chores like cleaning, cooking, and laundry.
- Companionship services: Offer social interaction and companionship.
- Skilled nursing care: Provides medical care, such as wound care, medication administration, and physical therapy.

Long-Term Care Facilities

When in-home care becomes insufficient, long-term care facilities offer various levels of support:

- Assisted living: Provides support with daily activities, medication management, and social engagement.
- Memory care units: Specialized facilities designed for individuals with dementia, offering secure environments and specialized care.
- Nursing homes: Offer comprehensive medical care and round-the-clock supervision for individuals with advanced dementia.

Part III: Caring for the Caregiver
Chapter 9: Practical Caregiving Strategies
9.3- In-Home and Long-Term Care Options

Factors to Consider
- Level of care needed: Assess the individual's current and anticipated needs.
- Financial resources: Evaluate the cost of different care options and explore potential funding sources.
- Personal preferences: Consider the individual's wishes and preferences for living arrangements.
- Caregiver well-being: Evaluate the impact of caregiving on family members and explore respite care options.

Transitioning Between Care Settings
As dementia progresses, it may be necessary to transition between care settings. This process can be challenging, but careful planning and communication can help minimize stress.
- Advance care planning: Discuss care preferences and create legal documents (e.g., power of attorney, living will).
- Involve the care team: Collaborate with healthcare providers and social workers.
- Visit potential facilities: Tour different care settings to compare options.
- Prepare the individual: Explain the transition in simple terms and provide reassurance.

Choosing the right care option is a personal decision that depends on individual circumstances. It's essential to weigh the benefits and drawbacks of each option carefully.

Part III: Caring for the Caregiver
Chapter 9: Practical Caregiving Strategies
9.4- Adapting to Daily Life Changes

As dementia progresses, daily routines and activities will inevitably change. Adapting to these changes requires flexibility, patience, and creativity.

Understanding the Challenges
- Increased dependence: The person with dementia may require more assistance with daily tasks.
- Changes in behavior: Mood swings, agitation, or wandering may become more frequent.
- Cognitive decline: Memory loss and difficulty with problem-solving can impact daily life.

Strategies for Adaptation
- Create a safe environment: Remove hazards and implement safety measures.
- Establish routines: Maintain consistent daily schedules to provide a sense of structure.
- Simplify tasks: Break down complex tasks into smaller, easier steps.
- Visual aids: Use pictures or labels to assist with daily activities.
- Adapt activities: Modify hobbies or interests to accommodate changing abilities.
- Encourage independence: Allow the person to maintain as much independence as possible.
- Seek professional help: Consider occupational therapy or physical therapy for assistance with daily living skills.

Part III: Caring for the Caregiver
Chapter 9: Practical Caregiving Strategies
9.4- Adapting to Daily Life Changes

Caregiver Well-being
- Prioritize self-care: Take breaks and engage in activities you enjoy.
- Build a support network: Connect with other caregivers for emotional support and practical advice.
- Seek professional help: Don't hesitate to consult a therapist or counselor.

Adapting to daily life changes can be challenging, but with patience, understanding, and the right support, it's possible to maintain a good quality of life for both the person with dementia and the caregiver.

Part III: Caring for the Caregiver
Chapter 9: Practical Caregiving Strategies
9.5- Managing Mood Swings

Mood swings are a common challenge for caregivers of individuals with dementia. Understanding the underlying causes and implementing effective strategies can help manage these fluctuations.

Understanding the Causes
- Physical discomfort: Pain, fatigue, or illness can trigger mood swings.
- Environmental factors: Changes in routine, noise, or overstimulation can contribute to irritability.
- Communication difficulties: Frustration with communication challenges can lead to mood swings.
- Medication side effects: Some medications may cause mood changes.

Strategies for Management
- Create a calm environment: Reduce noise and clutter to minimize overstimulation.
- Establish routines: Consistent daily routines can provide a sense of security.
- Communicate effectively: Use simple language, avoid arguments, and offer reassurance.
- Redirect attention: Distract the individual with a favorite activity or music.
- Physical comfort: Ensure the person is physically comfortable by addressing pain, hunger, or fatigue.
- Seek professional help: Consult with a healthcare provider or dementia specialist for guidance.

Part III: Caring for the Caregiver
Chapter 9: Practical Caregiving Strategies
9.5- Managing Mood Swings

Self-Care for Caregivers
- Practice self-care: Take breaks and engage in activities you enjoy.
- Build a support network: Connect with other caregivers for emotional support.
- Seek professional help: Consider counseling or therapy to manage stress.

Remember, patience and understanding are essential when dealing with mood swings. By implementing these strategies and seeking support, you can better manage these challenges and maintain a positive caregiving environment.

Part III: Caring for the Caregiver
Chapter 9: Practical Caregiving Strategies
9.6- Addressing Sleep Disturbances

Sleep disturbances are common in people with dementia. These disruptions can lead to increased agitation, confusion, and fatigue for both the person with dementia and the caregiver.

Understanding the Causes
- Disorientation: Confusion about time and place can lead to difficulty falling asleep.
- Restlessness: Physical discomfort or the need to move can disrupt sleep.
- Fear and anxiety: Worries about safety or unfamiliar surroundings can interfere with sleep.
- Medical conditions: Underlying health issues can contribute to sleep problems.
-

Strategies for Improving Sleep
- Create a sleep-conducive environment: Ensure the bedroom is quiet, dark, and cool.
- Establish a bedtime routine: Consistent sleep schedules can help regulate the body's internal clock.
- Limit daytime naps: Excessive napping can interfere with nighttime sleep.
- Physical activity: Regular exercise can improve sleep quality.
- Avoid stimulants: Limit caffeine and nicotine intake, especially in the evening.
- Manage pain: Address any underlying pain that may be disrupting sleep.
- Safety considerations: If wandering is a concern, consider using bed alarms or safety measures.

Part III: Caring for the Caregiver
Chapter 9: Practical Caregiving Strategies
9.6- Addressing Sleep Disturbances

When to Seek Professional Help

If sleep disturbances significantly impact the person's quality of life or safety, consult with a healthcare provider. They may recommend:
- Sleep studies: To identify underlying sleep disorders.
- Medications: In some cases, sleep aids may be prescribed.
- Consultations with a sleep specialist: For personalized guidance and treatment.

By implementing these strategies and seeking professional help when needed, you can improve sleep quality for both the person with dementia and yourself.

Part III: Caring for the Caregiver
Chapter 9: Practical Caregiving Strategies
9.7- Stress Management Techniques

Caregiving for someone with dementia can be incredibly demanding and stressful. It's essential to prioritize self-care to prevent burnout and maintain your own well-being.

Effective Stress Management Techniques
- Mindfulness and relaxation: Practice techniques like deep breathing, meditation, or yoga to reduce stress.
- Physical activity: Regular exercise can help manage stress and improve mood.
- Social connection: Spend time with friends and family to build a strong support network.
- Time management: Prioritize tasks and delegate when possible to reduce overwhelm.
- Seek professional help: Consider counseling or therapy to address emotional challenges.
- Respite care: Utilize respite services to take breaks from caregiving responsibilities.

Building a Support Network
- Connect with other caregivers: Share experiences and support with others facing similar challenges.
- Involve family and friends: Enlist their help with practical tasks or emotional support.
- Join support groups: Participate in local or online support groups to connect with others.

Remember, it's okay to ask for help and to prioritize your own well-being. By taking care of yourself, you'll be better equipped to care for your loved one with dementia.

Part III: Caring for the Caregiver
Chapter 9: Practical Caregiving Strategies
9.8- Managing Behavioral Challenges

Challenging behaviors can be a significant stressor for caregivers. It's essential to approach these situations with patience, understanding, and effective strategies.

Understanding the Underlying Causes
- Physical discomfort: Pain, fatigue, or medical conditions can trigger behavioral issues.
- Communication difficulties: Frustration with expressing needs can lead to agitation.
- Environmental factors: Changes in routine, noise, or overstimulation can contribute to challenging behaviors.
- Cognitive decline: Memory loss and confusion can lead to frustration and agitation.

Strategies for Managing Challenging Behaviors
- Remain calm: Your demeanor can influence the situation.
- Validate feelings: Acknowledge the person's emotions without enabling the behavior.
- Redirect attention: Distract the individual with a preferred activity or conversation.
- Establish routines: Consistent routines can provide a sense of security.
- Create a safe environment: Remove potential hazards and ensure the person's safety.
- Seek professional help: Consult with a healthcare provider or dementia specialist for guidance.

Part III: Caring for the Caregiver
Chapter 9: Practical Caregiving Strategies
9.8- Managing Behavioral Challenges

Specific Behaviors and Strategies
- Agitation: Identify triggers, provide a calm environment, and offer physical comfort.
- Wandering: Create a safe space, use alarms, and implement distraction techniques.
- Resistance to personal care: Approach with patience, offer choices, and provide privacy.
- Repetitive behaviors: Identify the underlying cause and find alternative activities.

Remember, each individual with dementia is unique, and what works for one person may not work for another. It's important to be patient, flexible, and willing to try different approaches.

Part IV: Additional Considerations
Chapter 10: Legal and Financial Planning

Effective legal and financial planning is crucial for individuals with dementia and their caregivers. It ensures that the person's wishes are respected, assets are protected, and future care needs are addressed.

Essential Legal Documents
- Power of Attorney: Appoints someone to make financial decisions on the person's behalf.
- Healthcare Power of Attorney: Designates someone to make healthcare decisions if the individual becomes incapacitated.
- Living Will: Outlines the individual's wishes for medical treatment in case of terminal illness or incapacity.
- Last Will and Testament: Specifies how assets should be distributed after death.
- Guardianship: If necessary, establishes legal guardianship for someone to make personal decisions.

Financial Planning
- Estate planning: Create a comprehensive estate plan, including wills, trusts, and beneficiary designations.
- Financial power of attorney: Grant someone authority to manage financial affairs.
- Review insurance policies: Assess the adequacy of health, long-term care, and life insurance coverage.
- Budgeting and financial management: Create a detailed budget and monitor expenses.
- Explore government benefits: Research potential government programs like Medicaid and Medicare.

Part IV: Additional Considerations
Chapter 10: Legal and Financial Planning

Challenges and Considerations
- Early planning: It's essential to address legal and financial matters early in the disease process.
- Capacity evaluation: Determine the individual's mental capacity to make decisions.
- Professional advice: Consult with an attorney and financial advisor for guidance.
- Ongoing review: Regularly review and update legal and financial documents.

Protecting Assets and Planning for Long-Term Care
- Asset protection: Consider options like trusts to protect assets from long-term care costs.
- Long-term care insurance: Evaluate the potential benefits and costs of this insurance.
- Medicaid eligibility: Understand the eligibility requirements for Medicaid long-term care benefits.

By taking proactive steps to address legal and financial matters, caregivers can alleviate stress and ensure the well-being of the person with dementia.

Part IV: Additional Considerations
Chapter 11: Effective Communication Strategies

Effective communication is essential for maintaining a positive relationship with a person living with dementia. It requires patience, understanding, and adapting to their changing communication abilities.

Understanding Communication Challenges
- Difficulty finding words: The person may struggle to express themselves.
- Misunderstanding: They may misinterpret information or have difficulty following conversations.
- Frustration: Communication challenges can lead to agitation and frustration.

Communication Strategies
- Simplify language: Use short, clear sentences and avoid complex vocabulary.
- Active listening: Give the person your full attention and avoid interrupting.
- Non-verbal cues: Use gestures, facial expressions, and touch to enhance communication.
- Visual aids: Employ pictures, objects, or written words to support understanding.
- Patience and empathy: Create a calm and supportive environment.
- Validate feelings: Acknowledge the person's emotions, even if you don't understand their perspective.
- Avoid arguments: Focus on understanding rather than being right.

Part IV: Additional Considerations
Chapter 11: Effective Communication Strategies

Specific Communication Techniques
- Repeating information: Repeat information in different ways to aid comprehension.
- One-on-one conversations: Reduce distractions by speaking privately.
- Using open-ended questions: Encourage the person to share their thoughts and feelings.
- Providing choices: Offer limited options to help with decision-making.

Tips for Caregivers
- Educate yourself: Learn about communication strategies for dementia.
- Practice patience: Avoid rushing or becoming frustrated.
- Seek support: Connect with other caregivers for advice and emotional support.

By implementing these strategies, you can improve communication and maintain a positive connection with the person with dementia.

Part IV: Additional Considerations
Chapter 12: The Importance of Respite Care

Respite care is essential for caregivers of individuals with dementia. It provides temporary relief, allowing caregivers to recharge and maintain their own well-being.

Benefits of Respite Care
- Prevents caregiver burnout: Regular breaks help to reduce stress and prevent physical and emotional exhaustion.
- Maintains caregiver health: Respite care allows caregivers to prioritize their own health and well-being.
- Enhances quality of care: A rested and refreshed caregiver is better equipped to provide optimal care.
- Provides social stimulation: Respite care offers opportunities for the person with dementia to interact with others.
- Facilitates planning: Respite care can be used as a trial period for long-term care options.

Types of Respite Care
- Informal respite: Enlisting help from family, friends, or neighbors.
- Formal respite: Utilizing professional caregivers or adult day care centers.

Part IV: Additional Considerations
Chapter 12: The Importance of Respite Care

Finding Respite Care
- Contact local agencies: Explore options offered by government agencies or community organizations.
- Inquire about insurance coverage: Some long-term care insurance policies may cover respite care.
- Support groups: Connect with other caregivers to share information about available resources.

Remember, seeking respite care is not a sign of weakness but a sign of strength and self-preservation. Prioritizing your well-being is essential for providing effective care.

Part IV: Additional Considerations
Chapter 13: End-of-Life Care and Planning

End-of-life care and planning are essential aspects of caring for someone with dementia. These conversations can be difficult, but they are crucial for ensuring the person's wishes are honored and for providing support to the family.

Understanding End-of-Life Care
- Palliative care: Focuses on relieving pain and suffering, improving quality of life, and providing emotional support.
- Hospice care: Provides specialized care for individuals with a terminal illness, focusing on comfort and dignity.

Advance Care Planning
- Living will: Outlines the person's wishes for medical treatment if they are unable to communicate.
- Healthcare power of attorney: Designates someone to make healthcare decisions on the person's behalf.
- Do-Not-Resuscitate (DNR) order: Specifies whether or not to perform CPR in case of cardiac arrest.
- Family meetings: Open and honest conversations with family members about end-of-life wishes.

Supporting the Caregiver
- Emotional support: Offer empathy and understanding.
- Practical assistance: Help with arrangements and decisions.
- Respite care: Provide opportunities for caregivers to rest and recharge.
- Grief counseling: Offer support for the grieving process.

Part IV: Additional Considerations
Chapter 13: End-of-Life Care and Planning

Hospice Care
- Pain management: Addressing physical discomfort.
- Emotional support: Providing comfort and companionship.
- Spiritual care: Offering spiritual guidance if desired.
- Bereavement support: Assisting the family through the grieving process.

End-of-life care is a complex and sensitive topic. It's important to approach these conversations with empathy, respect, and open communication.

www.ingramcontent.com/pod-product-compliance
Lightning Source LLC
Chambersburg PA
CBHW071837210526
45479CB00001B/179